SEA CHANGE

How Enhancing Vision Can Unlock Your Child's Full Potential

NICHOLA C. KENNEDY

FAOI mANBO

ISBN: 978-1-83556-357-1

TABLE OF CONTENTS

INTRODUCTION

As parents, we want our children to thrive academically, socially, and emotionally. However, sometimes we're left wondering why our child struggles with schoolwork, certain activities, or even following simple directions. The issues can feel like a mystery: Why is it that they can focus on a screen for hours but seem to fall apart when it comes to reading or homework? Why do they seem distracted, frustrated, or unmotivated?

The **good news** is, the cause of many of these struggles *might* be tied to how their visual system is working—or not working.

When you begin to understand the link between your child's visual struggles and their behaviour or academic challenges, it can lead to big changes. With the right strategies and understanding, not only can your child's struggles improve, but your entire family can experience less stress, more joy, and better communication. The changes you make to help your child thrive can transform your home into a more peaceful and supportive environment for everyone.

How To Use This Book: A Parent's Guide

In this book, we'll explore how your child's vision may be contributing to their challenges at school and at home. You've probably heard a lot of labels thrown around—dyslexia, dyspraxia, ADD, ADHD, or even "lazy" or "unmotivated." It's easy to feel bogged down by these labels, and as a parent, you may feel helpless trying to navigate them all. But often, a piece of the puzzle that isn't considered enough is how your child's eyes and brain work together.

What if their struggles weren't just about behavioural or learning issues, but about how they gather visual information? The connection between vision and learning isn't always obvious, but it can make a world of difference in how your child performs—and how they feel about themselves.

So, How Will This Book Help?

The Chapters: Each chapter will address a different sign or struggle your child might be facing, such as difficulty with focus, reading, or coordination. In each section, we'll discuss what might be going on in your child's visual system, why this could be causing frustration, and what you can do about it.

Reframes: You'll find 'reframes' throughout the book—new ways of thinking about what's happening. These reframes will help you see your child's struggles through a new lens, one that focuses on what's happening with their vision and how that affects their ability to perform tasks.

Actionable Tips: At the end of each chapter, we'll offer simple, practical tips to help you make a difference in your child's daily life. Whether it's breaking down tasks, using tricks to help them focus, or simply being more mindful of how they experience the world, these tips are designed to be easy to implement right away.

Standout Quotes and Examples: Each chapter also includes a standout quotes and examples to help capture the essence of what you're learning and make the key ideas stick. These quotes and examples are meant to be reminders of how vision plays a huge role in your child's behaviour, mood, and performance.

What's Next?

You're about to dive into an exploration of your child's visual system—an area that *might* hold the key to unlocking many of the struggles they face. By the end of this book, you'll have a deeper understanding of how vision impacts learning, behaviour, and emotional well-being, and you'll be equipped with simple strategies that can help your child thrive.

Let's begin the journey to understanding your child's vision—and how it can lead to a happier, more focused, and less stressful life for everyone in the family.

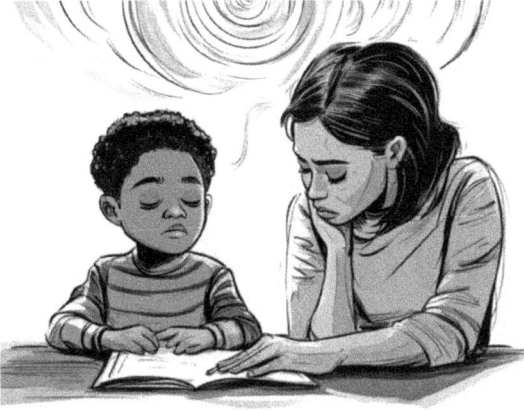

"Many children can focus perfectly on a screen for hours but seem to fall apart when it comes to reading or homework"

CHAPTER 1:

WHEN FOCUS FAILS – BUT ONLY WITH CERTAIN TASKS

As a parent, you may notice that your child can easily focus on some activities—video games, TV shows, or even conversations with friends—yet, when it comes time for schoolwork, they seem to lose focus or even start to struggle. They may become easily distracted, or frustrated, and avoid tasks like reading or writing altogether.

Reframe: This isn't inconsistency. It's a sign that the visual system can't keep up.

What's Going On?

When a child's eyes are struggling to process information clearly, it can lead to challenges with attention. The brain's ability to focus is tightly connected to how well the eyes are able to track and gather the information that they see. For example, tasks like reading, writing, or even simple homework assignments require a lot of visual effort. If the visual system isn't working as it should, focusing on these tasks can feel overwhelming to a child, causing them to "zone out" or become easily distracted.

What You Can Do

One way to make homework more manageable is to break it into shorter sessions—20 minutes at a time, with a break in between. This allows their eyes and brain to reset and stay fresh. Additionally, encourage your child to look far away every now and then, as focusing on something distant for a few moments helps reset their concentration. If the task is becoming overwhelming, you may need to step away, distract your child by changing tasks to something more active and then return to the work when they are calmer.

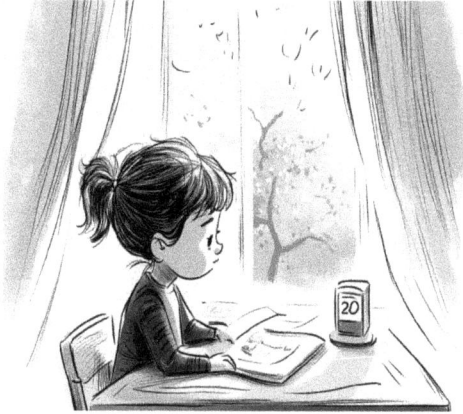

EMMA

Case Study: Emma's Focus Issue

Emma, 9, can focus for hours on video games and socialising, but struggles with homework. She's easily distracted and frustrated. After a vision check, it was found that Emma's eyes weren't able to keep up with close-up tasks. By breaking homework into 20-minute sessions with breaks, Emma's focus improved, and she was able to complete her assignments with less frustration.

"Tears, tantrums, or shutdowns over homework? You're not imagining it–and neither is your child."

CHAPTER 2:

THE HOMEWORK MELTDOWN LOOP

You know the drill—homework time starts with a sense of dread. Your child may put it off, get frustrated, or even cry before they've done much at all. You might see tears, tantrums, or even a complete shutdown.

Reframe: When near work overwhelms the eyes, frustration is inevitable.

What's Going On?

Visual fatigue can easily overwhelm a child's ability to focus on close-up work, like reading or writing. Tasks like homework often require sustained near-vision focus, which puts strain on the eyes. When the eyes aren't functioning efficiently—whether because of poor eye coordination, focusing issues, or visual stress—this task can become exhausting and frustrating, leading to emotional meltdowns.

What You Can Do

If your child seems to be in a constant state of frustration when it's time to sit down and do homework, try breaking up the work into smaller chunks. You can also encourage your child to look out the window or focus on something far away for a few moments to give their eyes and brain a chance to reset. And if the frustration gets too much, it's okay to step away for a little while. Return to the task once they are calmer. The **20:20:20 rule of visual hygiene** - every 20 minutes look 20 feet away from what you are doing (eg reading, homework, computer work), for 20 seconds. I like to add blink 20 times and that will help dry eye also! Then you can return to your work.

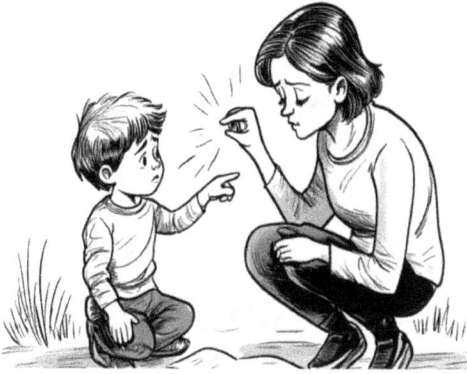

JOHN

Case Study: John's Meltdown

John, 7, often bursts into tears or tantrums when it's time for homework. His parents didn't understand why. It turned out John's visual system couldn't handle sustained close-up work. By splitting his homework into smaller chunks and giving him regular breaks, John was able to stay calm and finish his work.

"Your child is capable–
but poor eye coordination
can make them
seem inattentive."

CHAPTER 3:
LOST LINES & SKIPPED SENTENCES

Have you caught your child skipping lines while reading, or maybe they read the same sentence over and over without realising it? You might think they're simply not paying attention or aren't trying hard enough, but the problem could be their eyes.

Reframe: Their eyes aren't working together—but it can be fixed.

What's Going On?

When a child's eye muscles aren't properly aligned, they may struggle to maintain a steady gaze while reading. This means that while they're trying to read the words on the page, their eyes may wander or jump ahead, making it difficult to follow along. This isn't about laziness or a lack of intelligence—it's about poor eye coordination. Their eyes may not be working together efficiently, making it tough to stay on track.

What You Can Do

A simple trick to help your child stay focused on the line they're reading is to isolate that line with a ruler or a piece of card beneath it. You can also use a windowed ruler or even a strip of card to create a "window" over the line. This helps guide their eyes and keeps them from skipping ahead or losing their place.

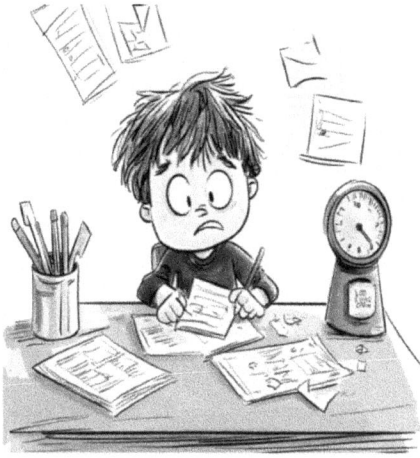

SARAH

Case Study: Sarah's Reading Trouble

Sarah, 8, would often skip lines or read sentences multiple times. Her teacher thought it was laziness, but it was actually poor eye coordination. Using a ruler to isolate the line she was reading, Sarah stayed on track and her reading improved significantly.

"Not every struggling child is disruptive. Some are quietly drowning, telling themselves they're dumb."

CHAPTER 4:

THE QUIET ONES WHO SLIP THROUGH

Some children may not show obvious signs of struggle. They don't throw tantrums or act out; instead, they quietly slip through the cracks. These children might be doing their best to keep up, but inside, they're silently frustrated and confused.

Reframe: Not all struggles are loud. Some children quietly believe they're not enough.

What's Going On?

Children who don't speak up about their difficulties may be silently battling visual challenges that aren't immediately obvious. They might struggle with focusing on the task at hand, or they could feel overwhelmed by the process of learning. This can cause them to fall behind, even though they appear "fine" on the surface.

What You Can Do

Don't assume that quiet children are thriving just because they don't show outward signs of distress. If you notice that your child seems withdrawn, frustrated with schoolwork, or avoiding reading or writing, it might be worth investigating whether their visual system is the issue. Supporting your child in a calm, non-judgmental way can make a big difference. Acknowledge their efforts, even when things don't go perfectly, and reassure them that their feelings are valid. Encouraging them during moments of frustration helps build their confidence and reminds them that you're in this together.

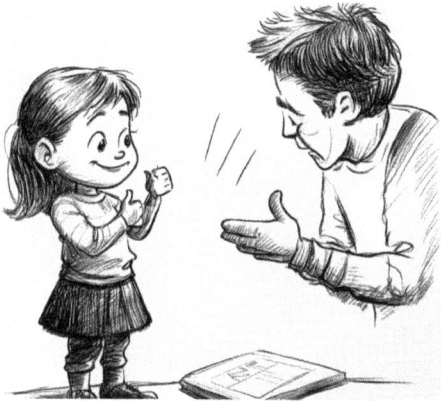

LILY

Case Study: Lily's Silent Struggle

Lily, 10, was quiet and withdrawn in class, and her grades were slipping. She struggled with reading but didn't ask for help. Her parents discovered her visual system was the issue. With targeted support at home, including visual aids, Lily began to thrive and engage more in class.

'Labelled as lazy, distracted, or defiant—but their head or eyes hurt and they don't know why'

CHAPTER 5:

WHEN 'BAD BEHAVIOUR' ISN'T BAD BEHAVIOUR

You may have noticed your child being labeled as lazy, distracted, or defiant. These labels can be frustrating for both you and your child, especially if they don't seem to match the child you know and love.

Reframe: What you're seeing is real. But the root cause might be hidden in their vision.

What's Going On?

When a child's visual system isn't working properly, they can act out, become distracted, or seem unmotivated—not because they want to, but because they're struggling with something they don't fully understand. Overloaded eyes and brain systems can lead to behavioural outbursts, lack of focus, or even resistance to tasks they find difficult.

What You Can Do

If your child is labeled as lazy or distracted but you know that's not the full story, try asking them how they're feeling in their body when these situations occur. Do they feel angry, frustrated, confused, or anxious? Are their eyes or head hurting? Understanding how your child experiences these struggles can give you insight into what they're going through. Supporting them in identifying what's causing their frustration can help you find ways to ease the tension.

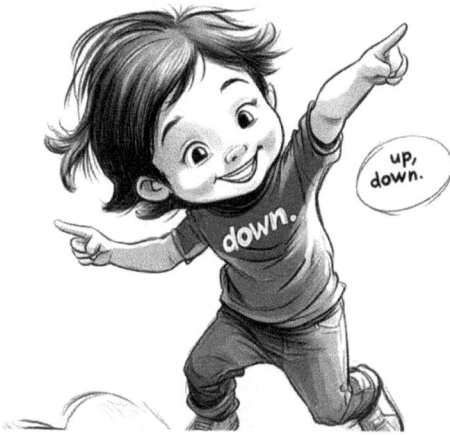

BEN

Case Study: Ben's Distraction

Ben, 6, was labeled lazy and distracted in school. But after a vision assessment, it was found that visual strain was causing his outbursts. With short breaks and tasks broken into smaller parts, Ben's behaviour improved, and his frustration decreased.

'Knowing right from left is more than just knowing which side: it's a foundation for understanding the world around them.'

CHAPTER 6:

RIGHT OR LEFT? THE STRUGGLE TO KNOW WHICH SIDE

You've probably noticed it—your child gets confused when asked to pick the 'right' or 'left' side. Maybe they hesitate during games or directions, or they can't remember which way is which. This is more common than you think.

Reframe: It's not about being careless. It's often a sign that their brain and eyes aren't fully in sync when it comes to understanding right and left.

What's Going On?

Knowing right from left seems like something that should come naturally, but it actually requires a lot of coordination between the brain, eyes, and body. When a child struggles with this, it's often due to difficulty with the visual system processing where things are in space. Understanding left and right is crucial for following directions, staying safe, and organising thoughts in tasks like reading, writing, and even physical activities.

What You Can Do

Developing the body's awareness of left and right through discovery experiences is essential. Go to the park or get out in your garden and figure out which hand can your child throw a ball further, which foot can they kick a ball further ?

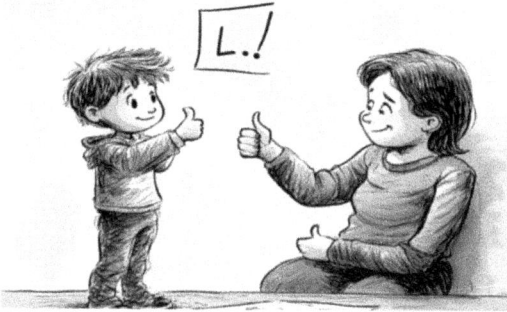

OLIVER

Case Study: Oliver's Direction Struggles

Oliver, 7, couldn't remember right from left, often confusing the two in games and class. His aunt taught him the "L" trick with his left hand, making it easier for him to differentiate right and left. This is a strategy however throwing and kicking a ball is a life skill which will help Oliver build more confidence in following directions.

'When direction gets confused, everything from reading to following instructions becomes a maze that's hard to navigate.'

CHAPTER 7:

DIRECTION CONFUSION – MORE THAN JUST MIXING UP LETTERS

Your child might have trouble with letters like 'b' and 'd' or struggle to tell if something is 'up' or 'down.' These are signs of directionality issues.

Reframe: It's not just a mistake. When the brain doesn't process direction clearly, it can make even simple tasks feel confusing.

What's Going On?

Directionality refers to understanding how things are oriented in space. Children who struggle with directionality often confuse left and right, up and down, or even words and letters that are mirror images of each other, like 'p' and 'q' or 'b' and 'd.' This can cause confusion when reading, writing, or following directions.

What You Can Do

A helpful trick for directionality confusion is to practice with large movement exercises. For example, having your child point to the sky when you say 'up,' or touch their toes when you say 'down.' You can also use visual aids like drawing arrows on a piece of paper and having them trace the directions to help solidify the concept of direction in their mind.

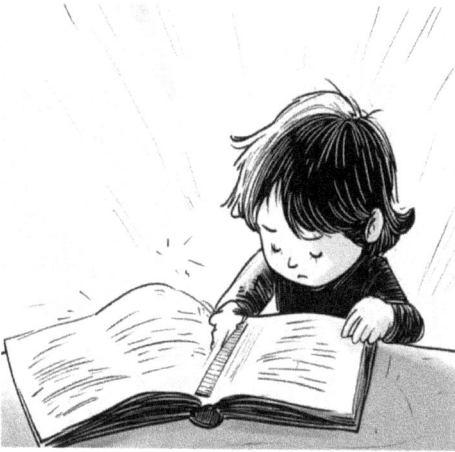

MIA

Case Study: Mia's Letter Reversals

Mia, 9, frequently confused letters like "b" and "d" and struggled with basic directional terms like "up" and "down." After practicing large movements (pointing to the sky for "up," touching toes for "down"), Mia's understanding of direction improved, helping her with reading and following directions.

'Clumsiness isn't just about being careless—it's a sign that the eyes, brain and body aren't syncing up to navigate the world.'

CHAPTER 8:

CLUMSINESS AND BALANCE PROBLEMS

Does your child trip over things, struggle with activities like riding a bike, or have trouble balancing?

Reframe: This isn't just clumsiness. It's connected to how their brain and eyes work together. When vision isn't working smoothly, balance and coordination are affected too.

What's Going On?

Vision plays a huge role in how we move and navigate the world. If a child's visual system isn't functioning properly, they may struggle with balance and coordination. This can make them seem clumsy, as their brain isn't getting the proper visual cues to control their movements effectively.

What You Can Do

Encourage your child to engage in activities that help them develop better balance and coordination. Simple exercises like hopping on one foot, walking in a straight line, or playing games that involve catching or throwing a ball can help improve their spatial awareness. Another simple hack is having them focus on an object across the room to help with tracking and depth perception. This encourages the eyes and body to work together more effectively.

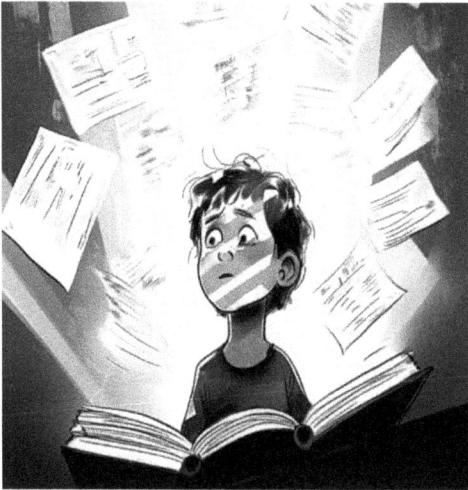

ETHAN

Case Study: Ethan's Clumsiness

Ethan, 6, was often called "clumsy" as he tripped and struggled with activities like riding a bike. After a vision assessment, it was found that his visual system wasn't helping with depth perception. Through balance exercises like hopping on one foot, Ethan gained better coordination and confidence in his physical activities.

CHAPTER 9
NEXT STEPS FOR YOUR CHILD'S SUCCESS

Now that you've gained valuable insights into how vision impacts your child's learning and behaviour, it's time to take the next step:

- **Get a Vision Assessment**

  If you suspect your child may be struggling with vision-related learning issues, consider scheduling an assessment with an optometrist who specialises in optometric vision training. A professional evaluation can uncover underlying issues that may be affecting your child's ability to learn.

- **Implement the Strategies**

  Start applying the simple tips and strategies you've learned in this book. Break tasks into manageable parts, incorporate visual exercises, and be patient as your child learns and grows.

- **Connect with Support**

  Share what you've learned with your child's teacher, caregivers, or other family members. The more people who understand the role of vision in your child's challenges, the better support they'll receive.

- **Keep Learning**

  This is just the beginning! Continue exploring the connection between vision and learning. Reach out to specialists, read more on the subject, and never hesitate to ask questions. Your child's journey to success is unique, and you're not alone in it.

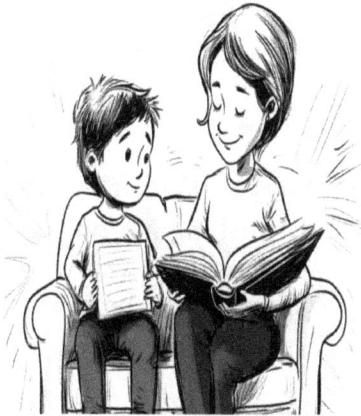

Remember: When the eyes and brain work together, your child's full potential can be unlocked!

ACKNOWLEDGMENTS

I would like to extend my deepest gratitude to all the families and children who have shared their experiences with me, and whose journeys inspired this book. Your strength, resilience, and commitment to finding solutions are at the heart of this work.

To the educators, specialists, and professionals who continue to guide and support children with learning challenges, thank you for your dedication and insight. Your work helps children see the world with new clarity.

A special thanks to Mary Grant, my business coach, for gently pushing me out of my comfort zone and seeing my vision even when I couldn't. Your guidance, support, and belief in me made all the difference.

A special mention to Robert Ledermann, who proofread my manuscript and provided honest feedback prior to printing—the power of LinkedIn connections!

And to my children, Jack and Chloe, who are my inspiration and gently guided me through motherhood and learning challenges. Your love, patience, and constant support are the foundation of everything I do.

Lastly, to my own family—my husband Robert, my parents Anne and Michael, and my parents-in-law Mary and Seamus—thank you for your unwavering support, encouragement, and love throughout this journey. This book wouldn't have been possible without you.

ABOUT THE AUTHOR

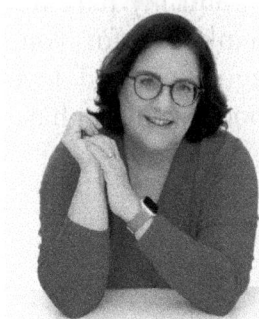

Nichola Kennedy FAOI mANBO, a **behavioural neurodevelopment optometrist**, is a dedicated advocate for children with learning challenges, specialising in the vital connection between optometry, vision training, and learning. With over 20 years of experience in this field, Nichola has helped many families understand how vision-related issues can impact learning, behaviour, and overall well-being. Through her work in **optometry & optometric vision training**, she empowers parents to recognise and address visual problems that may be hindering their child's ability to succeed in school and life.

As a mother of two children, Jack and Chloe, Nichola has personally experienced the challenges that learning difficulties can bring. Her children's struggles with focus and academic performance led her to explore the role of the visual system in learning. It was through **optometric vision training** that she discovered how significant a factor vision can be in a child's success. This sparked her passion for helping other parents navigate these challenges and inspired her to write *See the Change How Enhancing Vision Can Unlock Your Child's Full Potential.*

Nichola's expertise in **optometry and vision training** has led her to work with children facing a variety of learning difficulties, from dyslexia, dyspraxia, autism spectrum to ADHD. She believes that vision is far more than just seeing clearly—it plays a critical role in how the brain gathers visual information, and this connection is key to unlocking a child's full potential.

Outside of her professional work, Nichola enjoys travelling, spending time with her family, continuing her education in optometry and vision training, and advocating for a greater understanding of how vision and learning are interconnected.

Nichola lives in Co. Kildare, Ireland with her husband, children and their gorgeous golden doodle Buddy.

You can connect with Nichola online via her *website at* www.kilcullenoptician.com/brainsight *Intstagram* @kilcullenopticians & @brainsight.ie *LinkedIn* www.linkedin.com/in/brainsight

---

WHAT'S NEXT?

Thank you for reading *See the Change How Enhancing Vision Can Unlock Your Child's Full Potential.* I hope you've gained valuable insights to help your child thrive.

To continue your journey and stay connected, I invite you to visit my website and follow me on social media for additional resources, updates, and support:

- Website: www.brainsight.ie
  Explore more resources, articles, and information on optometric vision training and learning challenges.

- Instagram: @brainsight.ie
  Get practical tips and inspiration for supporting your child's vision and learning.

- LinkedIn: https://www.linkedin.com/in/
  brainsight/ Connect with me for professional insights, workshops, and further learning on vision and learning development.

Feel free to reach out with any questions or to share your child's story—I'd love to hear from you!

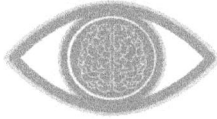

BRAINSIGHT ™

ENHANCE YOUR VISION
UNLOCK YOUR POTENTIAL

www.ingramcontent.com/pod-product-compliance
Ingram Content Group UK Ltd.
Pitfield, Milton Keynes, MK11 3LW, UK
UKHW042119120625
459614UK00006B/21